# The Home Workout Bible

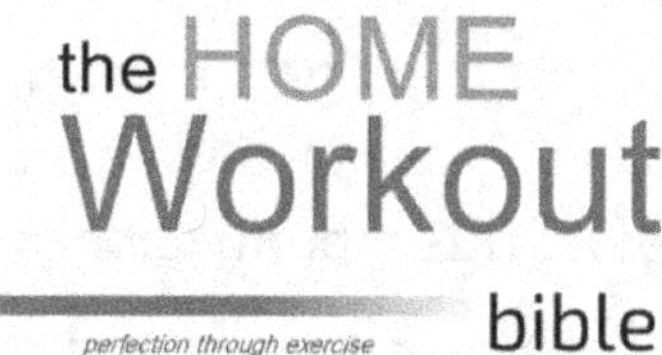



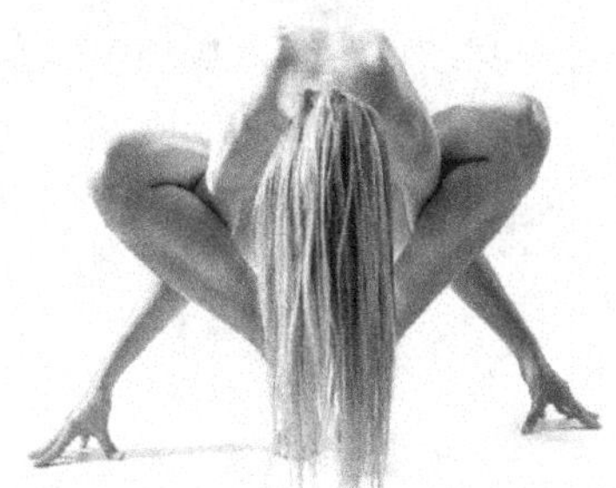

Phil Lancaster

get in the best shape of your life from home

# The Home Workout Bible

get in the best shape of your life from home

## Copyright and Enquiries

Copyright © 2025 by Phil Lancaster



Comments or enquiries may be left in the *Contact Us* page at

https://agingslowdown.com/contact-us/

# The Home Workout Bible

get in the best shape of your life from home

## Disclaimer

Please note the information contained within this document is for educational and entertainment purposes only. Every attempt has been made to provide accurate, up to date, reliable and complete information. No warranties of any kind are expressed or implied. Readers acknowledge that the author is not engaging in the rendering of legal, financial, medical or professional advice.

By reading this document, the reader agrees that under no circumstances is the author or publisher responsible for any losses, direct or indirect, which are incurred as a result of the use of information contained within this document, including, but not limited to, errors, omissions, or inaccuracies.

# The Home Workout Bible

get in the best shape of your life from home

## Contents

# The Home Workout Bible

get in the best shape of your life from home

# The Home Workout Bible



## Introduction

**N**o matter what your training goals may be, working out from home is almost certainly going to help you to get better results *right away*.

And in fact, if you're overweight or generally very *out* of shape, then I would argue that training from home is the *only* way to build muscle. Likewise, if your aim is to get into incredible superhero shape, then training from home is probably the only chance you realistically have.

Let's imagine for a moment that you're very overweight and you *really* want to get into decent shape. In this scenario, you will most likely have tried numerous different strategies to get into shape and you will possibly have been let down with the various workouts and diets you've tried. This is the tried and true story that so many people experience – they buy into countless supplements, countless weight loss programs, diets, training regimes... and they get nowhere.

But the problem isn't with the training programs. The problem isn't that they are somehow 'untrainable' and unable to achieve the shape they want. Rather, the problem is that they can't stick to the regimes and they don't manage to get to the gym *enough*.

Why? Because people who are overweight are usually tired. They're normally overweight because they're not active

# The Home Workout Bible



enough and they're not active enough because at the end of the day, when they get home from work, they have 3 hours before bed and they spend that crashed out on the couch. Small amounts of exertion make them sweaty and out of breath, meaning that they won't exactly *enjoy* training. Sticking to any training regime in this scenario is going to be hard – but when you add in the need to drive to the gym, then train in front of countless strangers feeling very self-conscious… is it any wonder it doesn't work out? Then you have to shower…

Compare this with training from home, which will allow you to slowly introduce small amounts of training into your regime, to increase your energy levels, your mood and your health. *Everyone* can fit 10 minutes into their day, especially when the equipment they need is right there and they can train in privacy. You see the difference?

But what about those real athlete types? These are the people with *no problem* generating the energy they need to train. People with *no problem* finding the will to train.

But with the best will in the world, even the top fitness fanatics on YouTube only have a finite amount of time in their day. There's only so much time they can spend training. If they're going to the gym every time they workout, then that means that they're going to be spending time and energy getting there – meaning there's less in the tank for their actual workouts!

# The Home Workout Bible



Then there's the fact that they have to wait for the equipment they want to train with to become free. Then there's the fact that there are some things you just can't do in the gym – some very basic things in fact.

Now imagine that you take a different approach and you build a home gym in your garage. Even if this is just a bench press, this is now a bench press you can use every single day. And this is a bench press that you can use whenever you want to without having to drive there or queue. Or maybe you need something more specific? Like a set of monkey bars you can use to do your own home street workouts.

Being able to train *whenever* you need to, with no queue and no drive. That's when you start to see truly incredible transformations. That's when you *truly* never skip a day at the gym.

So yes, training from home is the only way if you *really* want to smash your goals – no matter what they are. But of course there are some big challenges and some big questions that face those who want to start working out from home. Read on and let's take a closer look at how you can go about building muscles from home with programs that are guaranteed to work – and in some case get *incredible,* unheard of results.

# The Home Workout Bible

get in the best shape of your life from home

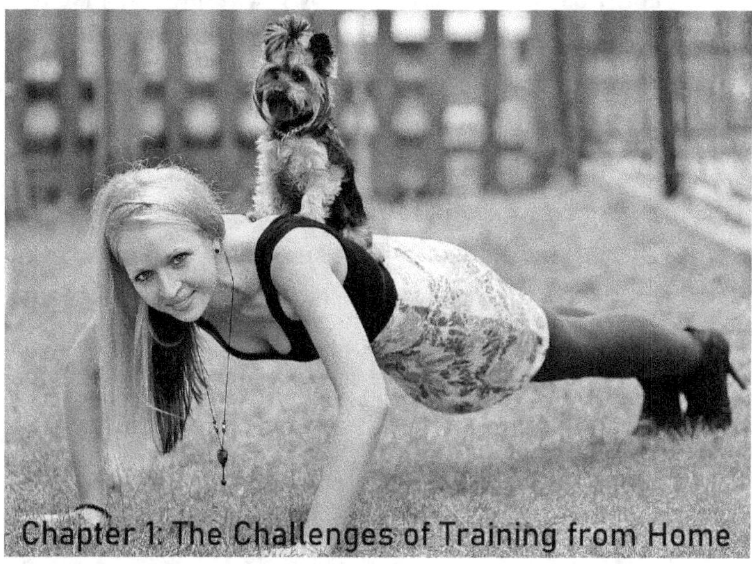



## Chapter 1: The Challenges of Training from Home

Gym managers are all too familiar with the New Year rush of gym memberships.

The majority sign up for a year, but quit after four weeks.

For all sorts of reasons. These include:

- I only need to FEEL as if I'm doing something positive. I achieved this by joining the gym and paying for the membership. I don't need to actually go as well.

# The Home Workout Bible



- Life has intervened. It's not my fault. I'm just too busy to go to the gym.
- I absolutely needed/deserved that glass/bottle of wine after the hellish day I've had. Now I've had too much to drink. I'll go to the gym tomorrow.
- I went to the gym, but it was full of all these people with great bodies who all seemed to know what they were doing. I felt totally intimidated, so I came home and poured myself a drink.
- My personal trainer created a program for me and I dived right into it. It was great. At the time. But now I feel like I'll never walk again. If working out makes you feel like this, then maybe it's not for me.

So what are the challenges of training from home? Surely nothing could be easier than staying in shape when you have a bench press *right there* in your own home?

Unfortunately, it's not that simple and there's a good reason that most people will start out by hitting a gym. The first challenge is simply stocking your home up with the equipment you can need. It is possible to get into great shape using only bodyweight training and we'll be discussing that in more detail later on. The thing is though, that in order to get fast muscle building results, training equipment *does* help. That then means dumbbells, pull up bars, bench presses, treadmills and all manner of others things – all of which cost a lot of money, take up a lot of space and require some basic knowledge to use.

# The Home Workout Bible


That's the other issue here too: knowledge. A lot of people simply don't know how to train on their own from home and this makes it remarkably difficult for them to build big muscle without going to a gym where they can meet trainers and see other people working out. Attempting a barbell on your own from the comfort of your own home can easily end up in a slipped disk or buckled knees! Fear is going to be immobilizing for a lot of people in this respect and prevent them from getting into shape.

And then there's the issue that a lot of people will have with motivation. If you're trying to get into shape in your front room, that means you have to try and avoid the distractions of TV and you need to stay motivated even though your bed is *right there*.

But even this isn't the hardest part…

## Pushing Yourself from Home

The problem, is that in order to build your strength or your fitness, you *really* need to be able to push yourself. If it's muscle you're trying to build, then that means you need to be able to create muscle tears and you need to pump your muscles with metabolites (more on this later!). This is much easier to do when you're lifting big heavy weights and then dropping down each time you reach failure. It's much easier when you have a trainer barking at you. And it's much easier when you're in a room filled with other people working hard, with no distractions and with a soft floor that you're fine to sweat on.

# The Home Workout Bible



The same also goes for losing weight. How do you lose weight? With lots of cardio. That cardio needs to be high volume, whether that is achieved through high intensity or long duration. Whether you're running for hours, or whether you're doing intense HIIT workouts – either way, training requires you to push yourself.

And when you're at home, you will often not know *how* to do this, nor be *able* to do it because you won't have the right equipment or necessary space.

But this book is here to change all that. In these chapters, you'll learn the secrets to training in such a way that you can break down muscle and transform your metabolism *quickly* and from the comfort of your home. Once you understand the logic, once you can crack the code, then you can go about building the power and health you're looking for.

So let's get started!

# The Home Workout Bible

get in the best shape of your life from home

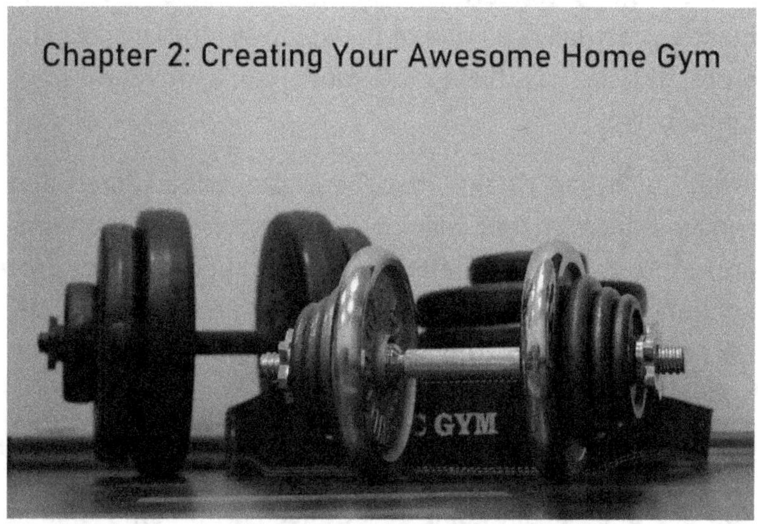


## Chapter 2: Creating Your Awesome Home Gym

To start with, you're going to need to create your own home gym. This means finding the right equipment and stocking up your home, whether that's a spare room, your living room or even a garage (which is just ideal!).

The exact equipment you're going to need is going to depend largely on the goals of your workouts and what you're trying to achieve. The equipment you need to burn calories and lose weight for instance, is quite different from what you would use to build *massive muscle*.

# The Home Workout Bible



As we're going to learn later in this book though, building muscle is actually still one of the key ways to burn fat. The more muscle you build, the more you'll drive up your metabolism.

What you'll find then is that there are certain things and certain principles that will apply no matter what your aims are. And there are definitely some specific pieces of equipment that everyone should own. Read on and let's take a look at what some of those are and how you should approach this process.

## What Makes a Good Home Gym?

You are once again going to be faced with some unique challenges here when you begin building your own home gym. The first of these is the simple fact that your home gym shouldn't cost too much. If you're relatively new to the gym and if you don't have any equipment yet, it can be tempting to stock yourself up with everything you think you might ever need and end up spending a small fortune.

Likewise, you need to think about how you're going to store your equipment. If you have a room dedicated to being your gym, then this latter point will be easy enough. But if you do not, then you need to think about how you can make a gym that will be easy to take apart and put back together on cue, or one that is simply small enough and compact enough that it doesn't matter too much.

Oh and you also need to make sure you aren't going to smash any cabinets or go through any tables.

# The Home Workout Bible

get in the best shape of your life from home

The best tip in this regard then is to start small and then build your way up. That means buying just a few items that you absolutely need to begin with but approaching them in a way that leaves you with the potential to expand and build upon that start.

Take dumbbells for example. Dumbbells are useful for practically every workout under the sun and can hit all manner of different body parts. But you're going to need dumbbells that are heavy enough if you hope to really make an impact on your muscle growth. Of course 'heavy enough' depends not only on your current progress (which will change with time) but also on the move you're doing. Lateral dumbbell raises are difficult to perform with anything above 10kg, even for a trained athlete. Conversely though, 10kg would be incredibly light for doing dumbbell presses.

So the way to approach this challenge is to start out with dumbbells that can be increased and decreased in size. This means you should be able to remove and add weights as the situation requires and as you build up. Normally, you can get dumbbell sets for around $30 that let you increase the weight up to 20kg. This is a great starting point, or you might want to buy *two* lots of dumbbells, which will then allow you to build up further still.

This is just one example of how you can approach your home gym in a modular and compact way if necessary, while at the same time saving money. Another example of something like this is the pull up bar. This is an incredibly

# The Home Workout Bible



unobtrusive item and one that will only cost you $10. You can even get pull up bars that don't need drilling into the ground – they will simply fit over the door frame in order to fix into place!

The best piece of equipment to upgrade your pull up bar? Gymnastic rings! Gymnastic rings are simply plastic rings that attach to rope and can be looped over a pull up bar. These then allow you to perform ring dips, muscle ups, the iron cross, reverse push ups (pull ups from a lower height, with your legs touching the floor stretched out in front of you) and all manner of other things! The best thing about gymnastic rings is that they cost very little once again and they can be stored in

A skipping rope meanwhile is a great alternative to a treadmill, while you can also do a surprising amount with a bull worker – a piece of metal that offers resistance when squeezed. As we'll see later on in this book, there are likewise *lots* of things you can do with everyday items from around the home!

So think a little outside the box, use these tips and the principles *behind* these tips and build yourself a gym that does everything you need it to without taking up all the space in your home!

## The Basics You Should Invest In

But for those looking for more specific instructions, the following is a good list of equipment that you can invest in over time to gradually build up your gym. Now note that none of these things are absolutely essential to get started *except* the pull up bar and *possibly* the dumbbells depending on your interests and goals.

Here is how to start...

## Pull Up Bar

As mentioned, a pull up bar is the bare minimum you need to start training and building muscle. The reason for this is that the majority of muscles can be trained using bodyweight alone. By performing press ups you can train the chest and the shoulders, by performing sit ups you can train the abs etc.

However, the parts that are hardest to train without equipment are the biceps and lats. These are 'pulling' muscles meaning you need to be pulling something in order to work them. Seeing as you can't pull the floor toward you, that means you either need to hang or curl.

Once you have a pull up bar, you can train your entire body – though it will be easier if you get a couple more items too.

## Dumbbells

Dumbbells are incredibly versatile and are used for much more than just bicep curls. They can also be used for all manner of presses, for triceps, for rows that work the lats etc. You can also use them to add weight to your body while you train your legs.

# The Home Workout Bible



Make sure to get dumbbells that can be increased in weight. Start with 20kg worth and buy two sets (giving you 40kg total) if you already have a good level of strength.

## Bench

If you want to take your training to the next level, then look at investing in a bench. This will allow you to use your dumbbells in a much more efficient manner in order to do dumbbell presses, flyes and all manner of other moves. The best bench will be one that has an adjustable back, this will mean you can sit on it *or* lie on it and that will in turn mean you can do isolation curls and other moves with it as well.

On top of this, look into getting yourself a bench that can fold up in order to be put away. This way, you can tuck your bench under a bed or behind a wardrobe and it doesn't have to get in your way as a result.

## Exercise Mat

This is not completely essential but you will find that training without an exercise mat can cause your floor to become slippery with sweat and can make a mess in your home. What's more is that a mat will make it easier for you to perform moves like sit ups without hurting your back or buttocks on the hard ground! This is also good for stretching and more.

## Skipping Rope

For simply burning calories on the spot, there are few things better than the simple skipping rope!

## Kettlebell

Now you're beginning to get more advanced. For training legs and burning calories, kettlebells are incredibly useful. That's because they will allow you to perform kettlebell swings and all manner of squats (such as goblet squats). This in turn will mean you can build leg strength without needing a bar to perform deadlifts and squats. That's good news, because performing deadlifts and squats requires a lot of space in your room and are expensive to set up. A kettlebell can also be used for all manner of functional strength exercises, including things like one armed presses.

## Gymnastic Rings

We already touched on the amazing benefits of gymnastic rings. The great thing is that these will let you do all the same exercises that TRX does but for a fraction of the price. In fact, they let you do a lot more seeing as TRX isn't really suitable for dips!

## Bench Press

For those that really want to get serious, a full bench press will eventually be a good investment. This will mean getting a bar as well, in which case you might want to move into permanent set up so that you aren't loading and unloading the bar every time you want to lift.

# The Home Workout Bible



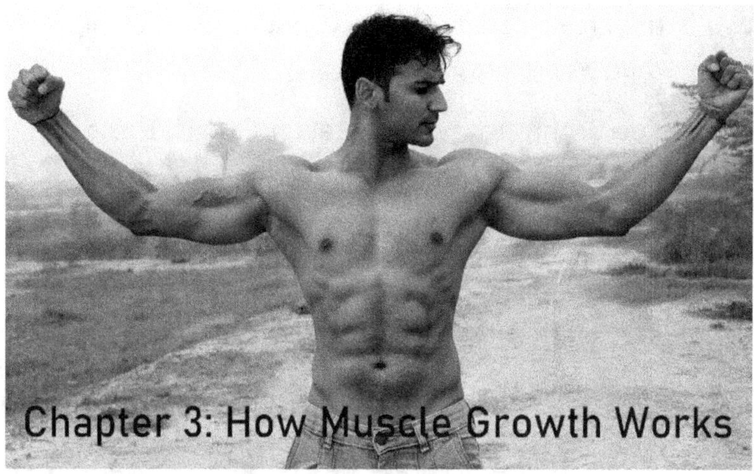


# Chapter 3: How Muscle Growth Works

Now you have the gym, it's time to learn how to use all that equipment in order to start triggering some serious growth. How to you get muscle to grow? How can you do this from the comfort of your own home with none of the hep or guidance you would get by working out in a real gym? Let's take a look...

## The Basics

In order to build muscle, you need to trigger hypertrophy. This is simply the technical term for muscle growth and it actually occurs when you're resting. This makes muscle building a 'two-part' process. Part one is the exercise that breaks down the muscle and marks it for growth and part

# The Home Workout Bible



two is the growth stage that occurs *after* you've finished lifting when you're at rest.

This can occur through two separate methods. These are:

Myofibrillar Hypertrophy

And

Sarcoplasmic Hypertrophy

The precise science behind these principles is still something that is being argued and there are those that deny that these are accurate descriptions. However, ask any bodybuilder and they'll tell you that broadly there are two ways to build muscle that seemingly correlate with these concepts.

Those two ways are:

Muscle Damage

And

Metabolic Stress

On top of that you have something else at play, which is the ability to build *strength*. Strength is often but not always related to muscle size. The other factor that is involved then and that you need to account for is:

Muscle Fiber Recruitment

Okay. So that's a lot of words I just threw at you. What does any of it mean?

# The Home Workout Bible



Simply put, your muscles are made up of lots of tiny strands called muscle fibers. These are actually cells, just like the cells that make up the rest of your body and the neurons that make up your brain. That means that they have nuclei and it means that they have sarcoplasm (if you remember enough of your high school biology…).

The difference is that muscle fibers have multiple nuclei and they also have the ability to telescope in order to contract and expand. Of course when this happens en-mass, it causes your muscles to contract and expand too, which is how you lift things in the gym.

Unfortunately, there is no way you can create *more* muscle fibers. This is known as 'hyperplasia' and has only been known to occur under very rare circumstances. However, what you can do is to break down the muscle in order to make it grow back thicker. You do this by lifting heavy weights to failure and especially under stretch, at which point you create 'microtears' in the muscle. Proteins are then used to repair those tears, which is what causes the muscles to come back larger. This is also what causes 'DOMS' – delayed onset muscle soreness. This is why you might find it hard to lift a mug of coffee the next day…

This is what we call **myofibrillar hypertrophy** and **muscle damage**. The most important factor here is to *overload the muscle*. There are other factors too though – such as making sure that you train the muscles from multiple angles to hit every fiber and training with both fast and slow form in order to train the fast twitch and slow twitch fibers.

# The Home Workout Bible



Fast twitch fibers only kick in when the slow twitch fibers aren't capable of lifting – and these are naturally the thickest and strongest types of fibers in your muscles. This is why you need at least a certain amount of weight in order to recruit them.

So what does sarcoplasmic hypertrophy involve? Well, this is muscle growth caused by swelling the muscles with fluids. When you lift for long enough, you gradually pump the muscles with blood and use up your lactic acid systems, filling them with those chemicals too. In other words, the part of your body that is working will start to become swollen with blood, nutrients, oxygen and energy. And if you keep on lifting, this causes that part of the muscle to become fuller and fuller and 'occludes' the area (like wrapping a tourniquet around it).

Now the good news is that all this also triggers the release of metabolites – chemicals that trigger growth such as growth hormone and testosterone. At the same time, the muscles become more efficient at storing sarcoplasm and glycogen in order to perform for long durations. This creates a more 'puffy' looking muscle that can perform for longer, rather than a harder and leaner muscle that can generate more short-term power.

So this is **sarcoplasmic hypertrophy** and it is caused predominantly by **metabolic stress**. The key factor in bringing this about is **time under tension** and it will lead to that feeling of *pump* in the gym.

# The Home Workout Bible



Both types are useful and when you combine both forms of training, you can build more size *and* power. As a general rule, bodybuilders tend to train more with sarcoplasmic methods, whereas powerlifters use more myofibrillar approaches.

Then there are those that say there can be no such thing as sarcoplasmic hypertrophy. It doesn't matter. Think of this just as a useful cognitive tool for understanding the process. At the end of the day, bodybuilders know that lifting heavy for small reps equates to more power, while lifting lighter for high reps equates to STRENGTH. Combining both is 'powerbuilding'.

Finally, there is one more concept we need to recognize here: muscle fiber recruitment. Because if you look at someone like Bruce Lee, you'll see that it *is* possible to be immensely strong without having to have a lot of muscle size. How? By using a higher percentage of your muscle fiber in every movement. Bruce Lee was the master of this but there are a number of ways you can train to gain more control over your muscle fiber.

The main key is to train at the very highest end of what you're capable of resistance wise. This forces your body to recruit as many of the fastest twitch fibers in the muscle as possible, which strengthens the 'neuromuscular junction' to increase your raw power output. Bruce Lee would even use a technique called static contraction, where he would push or pull against an immovable force to practice generating as much power as possible.

# The Home Workout Bible



Add this to your routine and you'll become even more deadly.

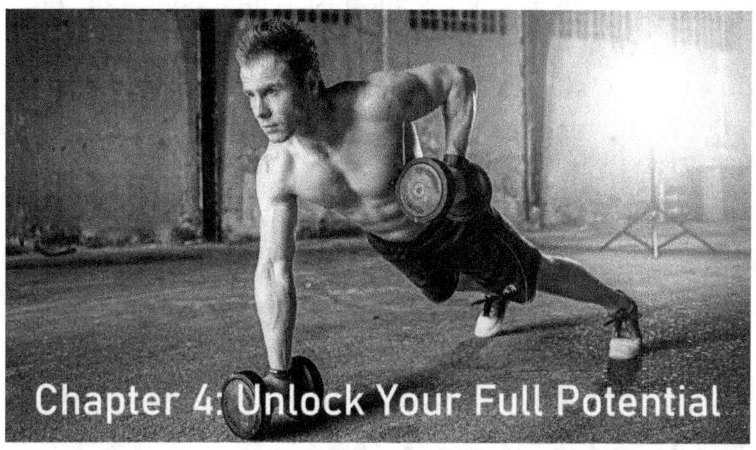


# Chapter 4: Unlock Your Full Potential

So now you understand how muscle growth works, you can start to apply this concept to your training at home. The key is to recognize that you need to create microtears, you need to create metabolic stress and you need to challenge yourself with increasing weights. You then need to ensure you get adequate rest and protein so that your body can build this back up.

This is where the discrepancy comes in with a lot of home workouts. Because if you are simply picking up a weight, curling it ten times and then putting it down, you aren't doing anything.

# The Home Workout Bible



All you're doing is using some fast twitch fiber and some slow twitch fiber to move a weight 10 times. You're building up a few metabolites and you're maybe causing a few tears – but it's not enough to see rapid growth.

You need to train like a bodybuilder.

What does that mean? It means you need to cause maximum stress and damage to the muscles and really challenge yourself. And that in turn means thinking outside the box and getting creative.

## The Weider Intensity Principles

The 70s are often referred to as the 'golden age' of bodybuilding. Back then, you had a lot of big names elevating the status of the sport, such as Arnold Schwarzenegger, Franco Columbu, Lou Ferrigno, Frank Zane, Sergio Oliva etc.

A lot of this popularity could be credited to media mogul Joe Weider, who observed these bodybuilders training and examined the techniques they used to trigger growth. He codified these to create the 'Weider Principles', which included such things as supersets, burns, forced reps etc. If you've ever trained with a fitness instructor, you may have come across some of these techniques!

At the time, Joe nor the bodybuilders he learned from necessarily understood the science behind these methods. Instead, they trained intuitively by listening to their bodies and starting to recognize the signs that a workout was working. But as it happens, all these techniques were either causing muscle tears or they were causing pump – and we can take some of these and apply them to our home workouts to make them much more effective.

In particular, I'm going to be looking at ONE of these techniques and then a variation on it. And it will change the way you train forever.

Seriously.

So the technique I'm talking about? That would be the *Drop Set*. A drop set is a routine where you start with a heavy weight, probably something you can lift for about 8-12 reps. You then perform your repetitions as normal until failure.

Then, when you've reached the point where you can't lift the weight once more, you simply lower it slightly and then carry on.

So let's say you're doing curls in a gym. You might use an approach called 'running the rack', which means you'll move down and down the rack until you reach the lightest weight. You might start with 15kg in each hand and perform 6-8 reps. Then you might put those down, immediately pick up 12kg weights and perform 5 reps. Then you'll put those down, pick up 10kg and perform 6 reps. Put them down, pick up 8kg and perform 5 reps. Then finish on 4kg and perform just 4 reps before collapsing.

That is *one* set. That means you need to repeat this whole process 3 times.

So why is this so good? Simple: it's causing the maximum amount of muscle damage AND it's swelling the muscle up with metabolites.

When you start out, you're lifting a heavy weight and you're going to perform 6-8 reps. This is as many reps as you can muster, so you're forced to engage a lot of muscle fiber, specifically the fast twitch kind which will exhaust quickly. Then, once those fast twitch fibers are exhausted and torn, your slower twitch fiber will kick in to help. Eventually, you won't have enough combined strength to keep going, at which point you can't lift the weight any more. Around the same time, you'll be switching from the ATP-PC system to the glycolytic system, which allows you to go for longer.

But you're not stopping at failure! You're picking up a slightly heavier weight and you're *continuing* to lift. This then allows you to engage your slow twitch fibers continuously while continuing to fatigue those few remaining fast twitch fibers that are still working, making even more microtears. At the same time, you're now reaching a much longer time under tension as you'll be approaching 20 reps. Your muscles will begin to fill up with lactic acid creating the 'burn' as a by-product of the glycogen energy system.

You eventually fail as a result but then you drop the weight and you *continue* to go – now relying entirely on slow twitch fiber and starting to tear those too – causing maximum muscle damage.

# The Home Workout Bible



Eventually it gets to the point where even 5kg is too much, at which point you've caused maximum damage that will lead to maximum growth of *all* types. It couldn't be more different from simply performing 10 reps of an exercise you can do comfortably!

## Applying This Method at Home

But this is difficult to do at home on your own unless you happen to own a whole bunch of weights and a rack you can move down. It's expensive, it takes up space and it's generally very difficult (though you can use a resistance machine!).

Instead then, let's take a look at a slightly different (and better) alternative. That alternative is the '**mechanical drop set**'. This is going to be the ULTIMATE tool for breaking down your muscle and for stimulating growth and most people still don't recognize just how powerful this technique is.

The idea with a mechanical drop set is simple: you can't make the weight easier to keep on going because adjusting dumbbells is limited and takes too long and because you don't own lots of weights.

So instead, you're going to change the *exercise* immediately and on the spot to one that is slightly easier. For example, you perform curls to failure and then swap to hammer curls (using a different grip) which makes them easier. Then you might move straight to chin ups (which works the biceps in a similar range of motion) and then to assisted chin ups (putting your feet on a chair). You've still managed to drop down four times and create one giant 'set' but much more quickly and with just one weight. What's more, is that you're hitting the muscle from lots of different angles to help create an even more 'all round' routine.

You can also insert some of Weider's other techniques as part of your mechanical drop set. 'Cheats' for example are exercises that you 'cheat' on by using momentum to get through them etc. For instance, you might swing your body in order to help with a curl. This isn't as good as a proper curl but as part of a drop set *following* proper curls, it works just great. Or you might perform burns – just barely moving the weight at the lowest point in the movement because that's all you can now do!

Use this technique to create 'circuits' and as an added bonus, the routine will be quite cardio intensive so as to generate more growth hormones and to help you burn some fat too.

## Putting it Into Practice

The other great thing about a mechanical drop set performed like a circuit? It allows you to fit in a lot more intensive training into a shorter amount of time.

This then allows you to use a very effective 'training split', which refers to the days you will train particular muscle groups. Specifically, the one we're going to be using is the 'push/pull/legs routine' or 'PPL'. This means you'll be alternating between push exercises (such as the press up and shoulder press), pull exercise (pull ups, bicep curls) and legs (squats, lunges, calf raises). These muscles are naturally complementary and breaking your workouts down like this will allow you to give each group enough focus to stimulate growth while also giving them ample time to recover subsequently.

Your routine might then look as follows:

Monday: Push

Tuesday: Pull

Wednesday: Legs

Thursday: Rest

Friday: Push

Saturday: Pull

Sunday: Legs

Or, if you are pushed for time, you can train just 3 times in the week.

## An Example

I'm not going to write down full workouts for you here for each and every body part – that's your job to come up with and it would be a waste of space as I don't know what your goals are or what your equipment is like. Instead, here is an example of what a workout for the pecs might look like performed at home:

# The Home Workout Bible

get in the best shape of your life from home

Push Routine

3 Rounds:

Pecs

6 x 20kg (each hand) dumbbell flyes on bench

8 x 20kg (each hand) dumbbell presses on bench

10 x ring dips

10 x clapping press ups

10 x rocking press ups (dipping down on each side)

20 x press ups

20 x press ups on knees

*2 minute rest*

Triceps

8 x 10kg tricep kickbacks

6 x 10kg dumbbell runners (slow motion running holding dumbbells and fully extending arms behind)

15 x rocking tricep dips (either side)

10 x tricep dips

5 x tricep bodyweight extensions

10 x tricep burns

*2 minute rest*

# The Home Workout Bible



Shoulders

8 x 20kg shoulder press

6 x 20kg incline dumbbell press (use a floor cushion to prop up your back if you don't have a bench)

5 x handstand press (using a wall if needed)

10 x decline press up

*2 minute rest*

# The Home Workout Bible

get in the best shape of your life from home

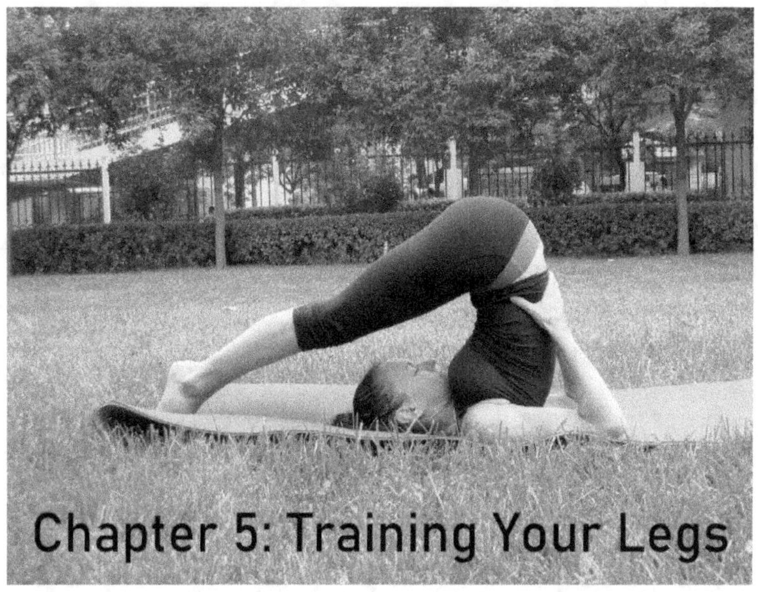



## Chapter 5: Training Your Legs

You can likely work out ways to introduce mechanical drop sets at home for your other body parts working around the weights you have. There are all manner of things you can do to make your exercises that little bit easier or harder and simply descending through these with no break will be enough to punish the muscle HARD.

For biceps as mentioned, you can go from curls, to hammer curls, to isometric holds, to pull ups. For lats you could progress from weighted pull ups, to pull ups, to assisted pull ups...

# The Home Workout Bible



But what if you want to train the legs? Things get a little more difficult here, so let's take a look at some ways around this challenging aspect of working out from home...

## Using Bodyweight

Using bodyweight, there are a few things you can do to train your legs. You of course have the regular squats, lunges and calf raises. However, these are likely *not* to be enough on their own to stimulate real growth.

In order to do this, you need to make sure you're involving the fast twitch muscle fibers. But your legs carry your body all day, so how do you make this harder?

One answer is just to get explosive. You see, your body doesn't see any difference between *weight* and *acceleration*. As far as your body is concerned, the exact same process is involved in moving something quickly as is involved in moving something heavy.

So instead of lifting a heavy weight with a squat, you can instead jump up onto a box. This will require activation of the fast twitch muscle fiber in just the same way to explode you upward. If you don't have a box to perform box jumps, then try jumping squats – these simply involve squatting and then adding a short jump at the top of the movement – it's perfect for building a little more power.

Another option is jump lunges – where you switch lunge in mid-air before landing. The calf jump is one of my favorites: here you jump by using only your tip-toes and not by bending your leg. This is also a great practice for building better jump height.

Alternatively, you can increase the challenge with bodyweight by increasing the relative force that you are exerting on each leg. The obvious way to do this? Stand on one leg! That way you can perform one legged squats and calf raises!

## Weighting Up

The easier way to do this though is to simply add weight using dumbbells and kettlebells. This way, you can mimic many of the big 'compound' lifts from the comfort of your home and with no need to invest in a barbell or a squat rack.

So one example of this would be to perform dumbbell clean and presses. Simply place a dumbbell by either side of you on the floor. Then squat down to the weights to pick them up, stand up with them, curl them up to your upper chest/shoulder and then press them up over your head.

Likewise, you can perform lunges which holding dumbbells in either arm. Or to make it more of a challenging whole body workout, try holding the dumbbells over your head, extended with fully straight arms.

Using a kettlebell meanwhile, you can start training in a manner very similar to training with a barbell. A kettlebell is a large round weight with a single handle protruding from the top. You can grab this handle with one or both hands and then pull it or swing it into position. You can also hold the kettlebell by the base with both hands in a bear-hug like manner. This can allow you to perform what is known as the 'goblet squat', where you squat with the weight resting across your upper chest. This move slightly moves the pressure compared with a regular squat – you're now working the quads slightly more than usual and the hamstrings slightly less than usual.

One of the best moves by far for leg training at home though is the kettlebell swing. Here, you grab the kettlebell in both hands and stand with your legs slightly apart and the weight hanging directly down in front of you between them. The object is now to swing the weight behind and through your legs and then up in front of you with straight arms. But you're *not* going to do this using your arms. Instead, you're going to do it by squatting down and then standing up and thrusting your hips slightly forward. The momentum alone causes the weight to swing up and then you squat back down as the weight comes down from the force of gravity. You don't break the momentum, you simply allow the weight to swing through your legs behind you and then thrust back upwards. Check out videos online to see how this works.

As you can see then, there are plenty of great ways you can train legs at home, so you don't need to spend a fortune on a squat rack!

# The Home Workout Bible



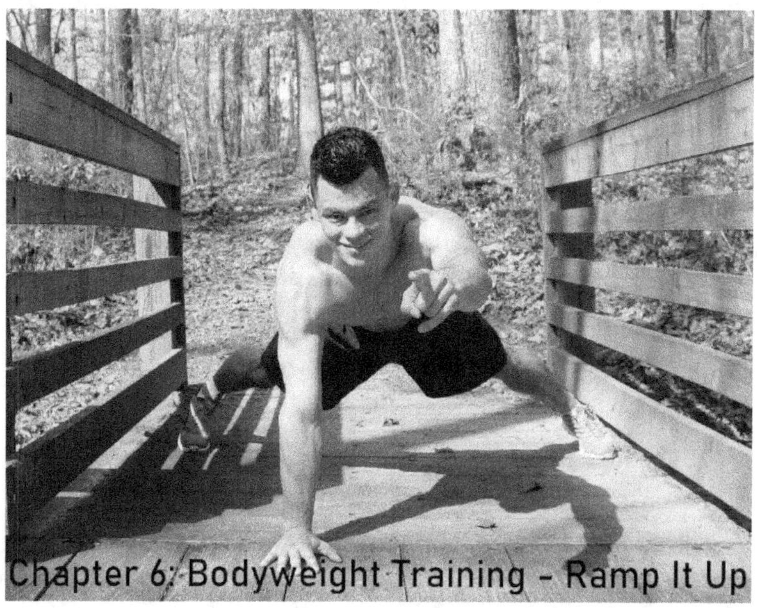


## Chapter 6: Bodyweight Training – Ramp It Up

One question I get a *lot* is whether or not you can build big muscle using only bodyweight training. Bodyweight training has a lot of appeal because it allows you to train literally from anywhere and using very little-to-no equipment. Bodyweight training of course incorporates press ups, sit ups, pull ups, chin ups, bodyweight squats and all manner of other exercises.

# The Home Workout Bible



But is this enough? Can you create enough resistance with *just* your bodyweight in order to challenge your muscles to grow?

Fortunately, the answer is a resounding yes – as long as you know what you're doing. And fortunately, you *do* know what you're doing because you have this book to hand!

## The Basics

The basic rule is just to make sure that you are creating that same damage and that same stress that we have been looking at so far in this book. It's not enough to just go through the motions, you truly need to challenge yourself. In the case of building muscle with bodyweight alone, that is still going to mean using the mechanical drop set. You can't increase the weight, so instead you need to increase the challenge by simply making the moves more difficult.

We've seen ways we can do this already: clapping press ups are harder than press ups for instance because they require more acceleration in order to get through the same movement. Then you have your one armed movements, which again create more challenge. You can also do something in-between a regular move and a one armed movement, by *rocking* from side to side. For instance, you might perform a regular press up but while dipping down slightly more on one side than the other. This will then allow you to keep the other hand in order to stabilize yourself and prevent yourself from falling but it *won't* be used to provide much of the actual strength and power needed to move through the repetitions. You can do the same thing with a pull up, chin up or tricep dip.

So now you have your obvious progressions for mechanical drop sets using only bodyweight: you can go from clapping press up, to rocking press up, to regular press ups. Or you can go from clapping chin ups, to rocking chin ups, to chin ups, to assisted chin ups.

Another option is to change the angle of your movement in order to alter the amount of pressure you're fighting against. This is referred to technically as 'extending the lever arm'. In other words, if you move the weight away from the point of contact with the ground, you're now going to make the movement more difficult. Similarly, you can make the move more difficult by reducing the number of points of contact with the ground.

So a press up can become a handstand press up, or it can become a Maltese press up with your hands down by your sides. Harder than either of these things is the *planche* where you're going to be holding your body parallel with the floor by just your hands: like a press up without your feet touching the floor!

Some of these movements are incredibly difficult. Not only do they require a lot of power in the target muscles, they also require tons of functional strength: you need to be able to coordinate and control all the muscles in your body to work together. That means making your core tight enough to stabilize your body and it means making your forearms and hands strong enough to balance you in a handstand. It means having enough control over your legs in order to keep them upright.

These advanced moves then become entire full-body exercises each of them. These aren't *as* useful for growing specific muscles because they don't 'isolate' a target muscle. That means it's harder to exhaust or tear muscle fibers in any particular muscle because there are too *many* points of failure.

But if performance is your interest, then this is an incredibly useful way to train. And if you use the moves as part of a mechanical drop set, then likewise they become powerful tools to help you exhaust the fast twitch muscle fibers first before moving onto easier moves to flood the muscles with blood and metabolites.

## How to Perform Awesome Beast Moves

Once you can accomplish these more advanced moves then, you start to open up a lot of new possibilities and to be able to create incredibly challenging workouts wherever you are. That and they just *look* awesome – like incredibly party tricks. If you want to train to make other people stand up and take notice, then this is sure one way to accomplish that!

The only problem? These really *are* advanced moves. To add these to your routines you're going to need an awful lot of power to begin with in order to perform them. So how do you get yourself to that point?

# The Home Workout Bible

get in the best shape of your life from home

Let's take a look...

## Break it Down

The problem here is that the jump from a press up to a handstand press up is so great, that you're going to have an incredibly hard time building up to it. 200 press ups still don't prepare you for a handstand press up, neither does a decline press up. So what can you do?

The answer is to try and break down those bigger moves into smaller components that you can challenge yourself with. So a good place to start would be with a frog stand – perch yourself just on your two hands with your knees by your elbows and balance there. Then try and just do presses like that. Then try and progress from that position to a handstand position with your legs tucked in. As you can see, making these into smaller steps means you can get closer and see yourself progressing more closely.

The next tip is to make sure that you really *focus* on what all your muscles are doing at the time. This training is not just for your muscles – it's for your brain as well. Specifically, it is for your motor cortex to learn the technique necessary to perform these moves.

Now let's take a brief interlude and think about a situation where our brain is fantastic at learning: during computer games!

When you play a computer game, you'll be focussing on the game so much that your skill will improve rapidly. Some people can pull off *incredible* feats in games after not that long playing. What happens here is that they watch the game and they anticipate and visualize the movement they want to perform in the game. They then try and do it and if they get it right, their brain rewards them with a flood of hormones including dopamine and others that help to cement the neural connections that lead to that movement. The more they repeat this, the more those connections are strengthened and each time the game rewards them with a chime sound or victorious music, that only strengthens this effect and makes them feel even more accomplished! When things go wrong, they lose health, the screen flashes red and there are very clear cues that this was the wrong move. Thus the brain doesn't get that response and the movement is not enforced. But really, that sense of reward comes from the fact that they so badly want to succeed. It comes from the fact that they are incredibly focussed on what they're doing and that they feel real anxiety and stress as they play and their health whittles down.

We can learn *anything* if we approach it in a similar manner. In the case of working out, that means setting real goals for yourself – to transition into handstand with perfect technique – and then paying close attention to the outcome of your attempt. Was that right or wrong? Should it be enforced or not? The more you focus on that muscle, the quicker you're adapt and your brain will learn how to pull off the perfect technique!

# The Home Workout Bible



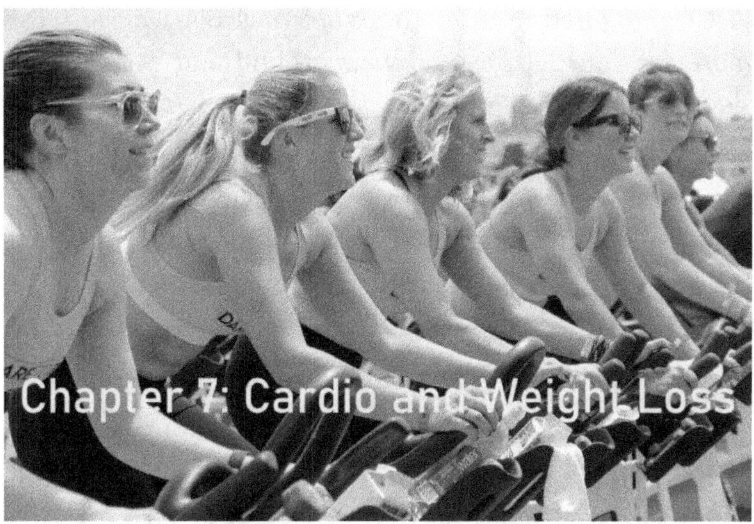


## Chapter 7: Cardio and Weight Loss

This is all well and good but perhaps you're wondering if any of what we've discussed so far applies to you…

Specifically, if your objective is to lose weight, then what use is the bench press? Or any of Joe Weider's other principles for triggering mass muscle growth?

Actually, everything! If you want to lose weight, then one of the very best things you can do is to train with weights. Not only does this burn a lot of calories and carbs in its own right but it will also help to change your metabolism and help you to burn even more fat even as you're resting. This is simply because it takes a certain amount of energy for the body just to *maintain* muscle. The more muscular you are, the more fat you burn as you walk around and even as you sleep!

What's more, is that muscle helps you to appear more toned and athletic. This is a big factor for a lot of people and is actually often more important than weight loss. Let's say for example that you have excess cellulite on your legs: should you burn calories or tone muscle? The answer is tone muscle, which will be *far* more effective at removing the appearance of the cellulite and helping you to look leaner.

A lot of women shy away from resistance training because they think it's going to make them suddenly appear muscular and manly. Even some guys will shy away from it because they don't want to look 'too big'.

But in reality, it is actually very hard to get to the point that a lot of people think of as 'too big'. No one *accidentally* ended up looking like Arnold Schwarzenegger – it takes a lot of hard work to build that much muscle. And as for women, lifting weights is one of the best ways to get a toned, feminine physique. Just try searching 'women who lift' in Google to see what I mean…

In order to bring about these impressive weight loss changes, you need to do more compound exercises in particular. These are the ones that utilize the entire body – so those bodyweight moves and also things like the kettlebell swing. The kettlebell swing will use the shoulders, the legs, the core, the back and more and that makes it an incredible tool for burning calories and building muscle.

## Adding CV Work

But what the kettlebell swing *also* is, is an example of cardiovascular training. The fact that you're swinging a kettlebell means that you're maintaining a high and consistent level of exertion. This allows you to burn calories but because you're using muscle at the same time to shift such a lot of weight, you're burning even more muscle and flooding the body with growth hormone as well.

In this way, you can use kettlebells like running and maintain output to burn lots of calories. The difference? A) you're working harder because there's weight involved B) this also prevents the body from catabolizing the muscle and C) you'll be able to do it from the comfort of your own home!

Perform 200 kettlebell swings and you'll burn a LOT while at the same time building up a lot of strength. This is especially true if you accomplish it using a drop set, so that you can start with a hard weight.

### HIIT

Another way you can take this even further is to use the kettlebell as part of a HIIT program. HIIT stands for 'High Intensity Interval Training'. This means that you're going to be exerting yourself 100% for short durations, then taking brief spells of rest in-between by performing at a lower intensity. So you might swing the kettlebell for 1 minute at

# The Home Workout Bible



full-power, then stop to jog lightly on the spot for 2 minutes, then return to swinging the kettlebell.

This allows you to burn more calories in a shorter amount of time than regular 'steady state' cardiovascular exercise. Better yet, it has also been shown in studies to help increase your mitochondria – the energy factories in your cells that allow you to exert yourself for long periods.

But the real power of HIIT lies in the way it helps you to burn more calories *subsequently*. That's because going at 100% exertion (that's 90%+ of your max heart rate) causes the body to work faster than it can get energy from your fat stores. This is called 'anaerobic training' and it forces the body to rely on energy stored in the muscles and the blood. When it does this, that then means that when you perform the slower exercise in-between, you *only* have the fat stores to draw on. So ironically, this means you end up burning much *more* fat in the long term. This process then continues even once you've finished training and you begin going about your regular business.

Using 10 minutes of HIIT a day, you can nicely cut off any fat you're worried about and increase your calorie burn. This is recommended as part of a 'finisher' – a routine you use to cap off a resistance workout and to increase your overall calorie burn.

# The Home Workout Bible



## In Defence of Steady State Cardio

But that said, you shouldn't write off steady state cardio just yet – be that performing 200 kettlebell swings, going for a 5 mile run, or just skipping for an hour.

When you do this, you will burn a LOT of calories due to the sheer amount of time – and this will certainly be more than you'll get from 10 minutes of HIIT. Think of HIIT as being useful when you want to work out in a shorter amount of time – it's more efficient, but you can only keep it up so long. It's also brutal and not for beginners.

The other benefit of steady state though is what it does for your general fitness and your energy levels. If you can maintain exertion throughout a steady state workout, then you will be taxing your heart a lot. This is good because it will allow the left ventricle to enlarge, just as any other muscle responds to training.

When *that* happens, it means that you'll be able to move more blood around the body with each pump. This is very important because it means in turn that you'll be able to more efficiently deliver blood, nutrients and oxygen to the muscles. It also means that when you're not training, your resting heart rate will be lower. This can actually benefit hypertrophy when you're resting and it will help you to sleep far more efficiently so that you wake up feeling more rested and better able to tackle the day ahead – workout and all!

# The Home Workout Bible



Just running 5 miles a week is more than enough to see your resting heartrate and your VO2 max improve. This will not only burn a lot of calories but it will also help to support an active lifestyle and especially when it comes to training. This is recommended for everyone.

But if you want to lose more weight, then you can of course increase the ratio of CV to lifting. That might mean that you add in lots of HIIT sessions, or it might mean that you maintain your steady state for much longer. Either way, this will make more sense in the next chapter...

# The Home Workout Bible



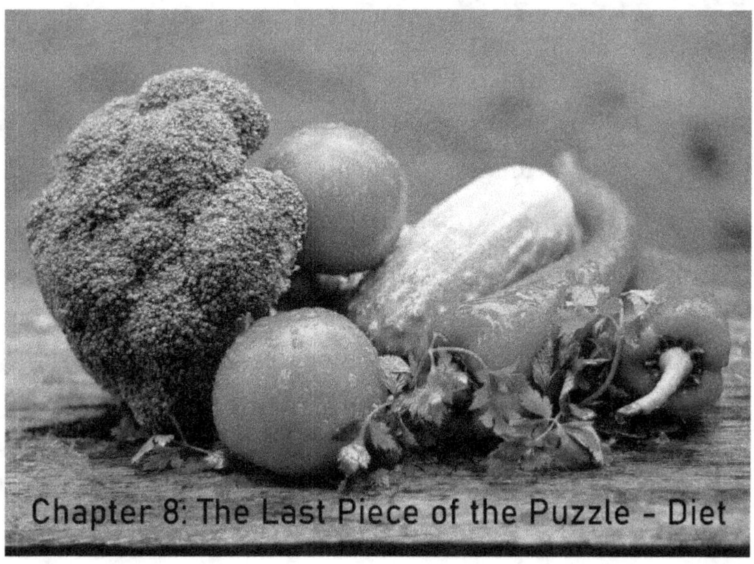


# Chapter 8: The Last Piece of the Puzzle – Diet

Finally, you need to think about the final piece of puzzle: the diet. Because whether you're working out at home or in the gym, your diet is one of the MOST important factors for ensuring the maximum benefit from your training.

Likewise, diet is crucial whether you want to lose weight or build muscle – though the strategy will change.

# The Home Workout Bible



## Calories VS Carbs

Unfortunately though, while diet is the same no matter where you're training, it's also not all that simple. Specifically, there is a lot of argument regarding diet and views on the matter can broadly be split into two camps.

On the one hand, you have the group that claim 'a calorie is a calorie'. Their belief is that the only factor that matters when it comes to losing weight, is the number of calories coming in and the number of calories going out. If you track all your calories, you then simply have to make sure that you burn off more than you consume and you'll lose weight.

This makes sense, seeing as excess calories are stored as fat and when you have a calorie *deficit* the body has to burn fat to get more.

So how do you eat a diet to support weight loss according to this idea? Simple: you calculate how many calories you burn in a day (by wearing a fitness tracker, or by calculating your active metabolic rate) and then you make sure that you eat less than that. To build muscle conversely, your objective is to eat a lot of protein which the body can convert into muscle and to be in a caloric *surplus* so that you have extra fuel to use for growth.

But then there's the other school of thought. This looks more at the way calories are used at different times. After training for instance, calories are more likely to be used to refuel glycogen. Likewise, some people will have different hormone balances than others, which will impact the way they burn fat. That's why some people never seem to lose weight and others never seem to gain it. These people recommend avoiding carbs and eating a diet rich in fats and proteins. This will support muscle growth, while the lack of carbs will prevent insulin spikes which can lead to fat storage. For building muscle, consuming lots of calories is important because you need insulin to build muscle and low calorie diets stimulate the release of myostatin – which breaks down muscle.

A calorie is not a calorie according to this crowd. More important is to avoid simple carbs and to eat nutritious meals at the right time, while maintaining a consistent blood sugar.

## The Answer

So who is right?

Well, both groups of course.

Maintaining a lower caloric intake than your daily burn *will* always lead to weight loss. The caveat is that you can never calculate how much you're burning accurately. Why? Because the amount of calories you burn is dependent on your metabolism – which has to do with a range of factors, including things like blood sugar and testosterone.

You can't deny the role of hormones: otherwise steroids wouldn't make people become ripped machines and hypothyroidism wouldn't cause people to lose weight.

The trick is to eat below your *estimated* AMR, while at the same time doing everything you can to encourage your body's metabolism. Actually the best way to do that, is to make sure that you're eating nutritious, natural and healthy foods, while at the same time working out and lifting muscle. Remember: building muscle MAKES you burn more fat, even when you're resting. That's why running and using resistance training is *so* good for creating a lean and toned physique and when you combine this with the right diet, you are attacking your fitness and your health on all fronts.

The hard part is just putting this into practice. Monitoring all the calories coming in and out of your body takes a long time and is rather joyless, so for most people it will be sufficient to make a strong estimate instead. Likewise, you can make life easier for yourself if you eat a relatively consistent breakfast and lunch. If you do that, then you'll be able to avoid having to calculate how many calories are in those meals on most days – it will be enough to just guestimate how much is in your dinner and then add that to the total. Maintaining a consistent breakfast and lunch is much easier because these are functional rather than social meals – we tend to eat them when we're on our own rather than out with friends.

## Conclusion

And with that, you now know everything you need to know to build muscle, lose weight and transform your shape from home.

# The Home Workout Bible



Hopefully, the main thing you've learned is what it is that makes a workout effective. A lot of us find that our workouts at the gym are more effective but we aren't sure why. The answer is that we're able to really push ourselves: to cause massive damage to our muscle tissue and to trigger a large amount of metabolic stress. When we get home, we end up just going through the motions and don't manage to cause this same damage.

But when you understand what it takes to make a workout effective – the methodical breakdown of muscle tissue, the flooding of metabolites and the continuous exertion – then you learn how you can employ the same methods no matter where you are or what equipment you're using!

And once you can train from home, you can train at your very hardest, any time of day. That's when you start to see *incredible* transformations.

# The Home Workout Bible
get in the best shape of your life from home

## The Rest of the Books

### The Series

The Home Workout Bible is Book 6 in the Fitness Blueprint series:

1. New Year Detox
2. Clean Eating for Weight Loss
3. Beginner's Keto
4. 4 Minute Keto
5. Keto Diet + Intermittent Fasting
6. The Home Workout Bible

Each book can be read stand-alone, but as a series they lead you through a journey, starting with a detox, then learning clean eating and proceeding to the keto diet and exercise to burn fat and become the best you can be.

See the full series at Fitness Blueprint on Amazon.

### Other Books

To see all of this author's books, both published and forthcoming titles and to get some free gifts, please sign up at:

https://agingslowdown.com/stay-informed/

# The Home Workout Bible

get in the best shape of your life from home

## About the Author

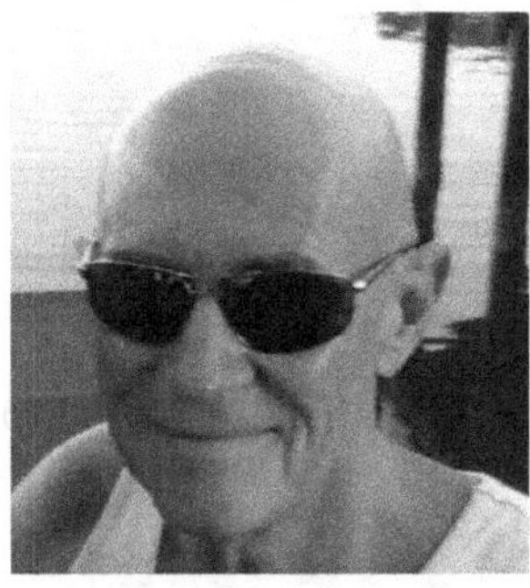

Phil Lancaster is an 80 year old (in 2024) Australian who embraces the Clean Eating and Fitness lifestyle.

He can do 110 pushups without stopping, hold a 5 minute plank, bench press more than his own bodyweight and does 100 km (about 65 miles) bike rides for fun. He weighs the same as he did when he was 18.

He literally never gets a cold or the flu. Not ever. Or hay fever, sniffles, coughing fits or asthma. Or back pain.

And he is a zero contributor to Big Pharma's bottom line.

That's right. He spends nothing on drugs.

No prescribed drugs and no over the counter drugs. He believes that all drugs have undesirable side effects and that most of your medicinal needs can be satisfied by eating the right food and priming your body's natural ability to fight disease and keep you healthy.

He believes that anyone can do the same. You just need to follow the blueprint.

He has 4 children and 4 grandchildren (aged from 15 to 25 years old in 2024) and intends to watch them all grow up.

www.ingramcontent.com/pod-product-compliance
Lightning Source LLC
Chambersburg PA
CBHW061524250726
48657CB00005B/2072